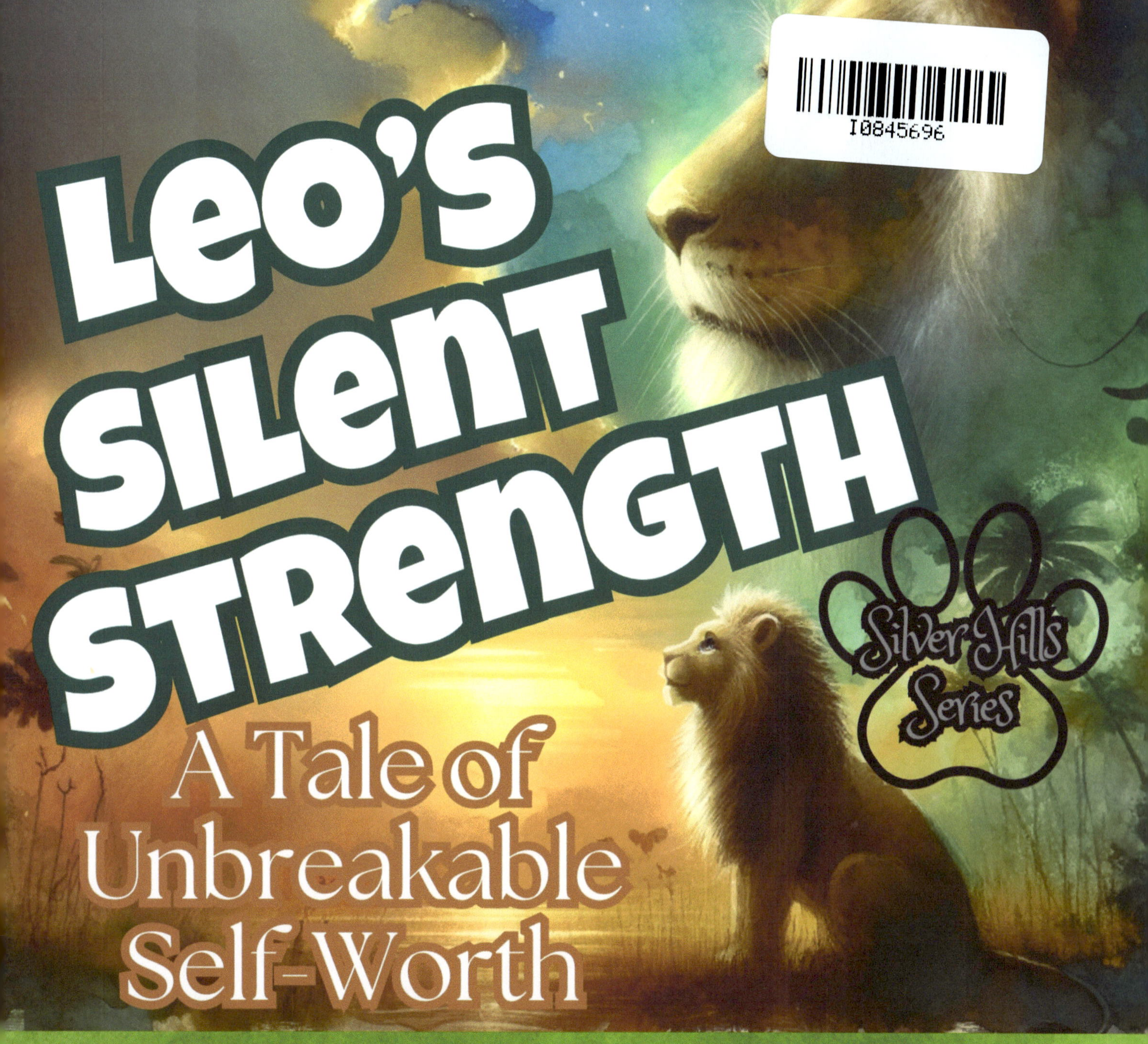

LEO'S SILENT STRENGTH

A Tale of Unbreakable Self-Worth

Silver Hills Series

Creative Adventures, TKM

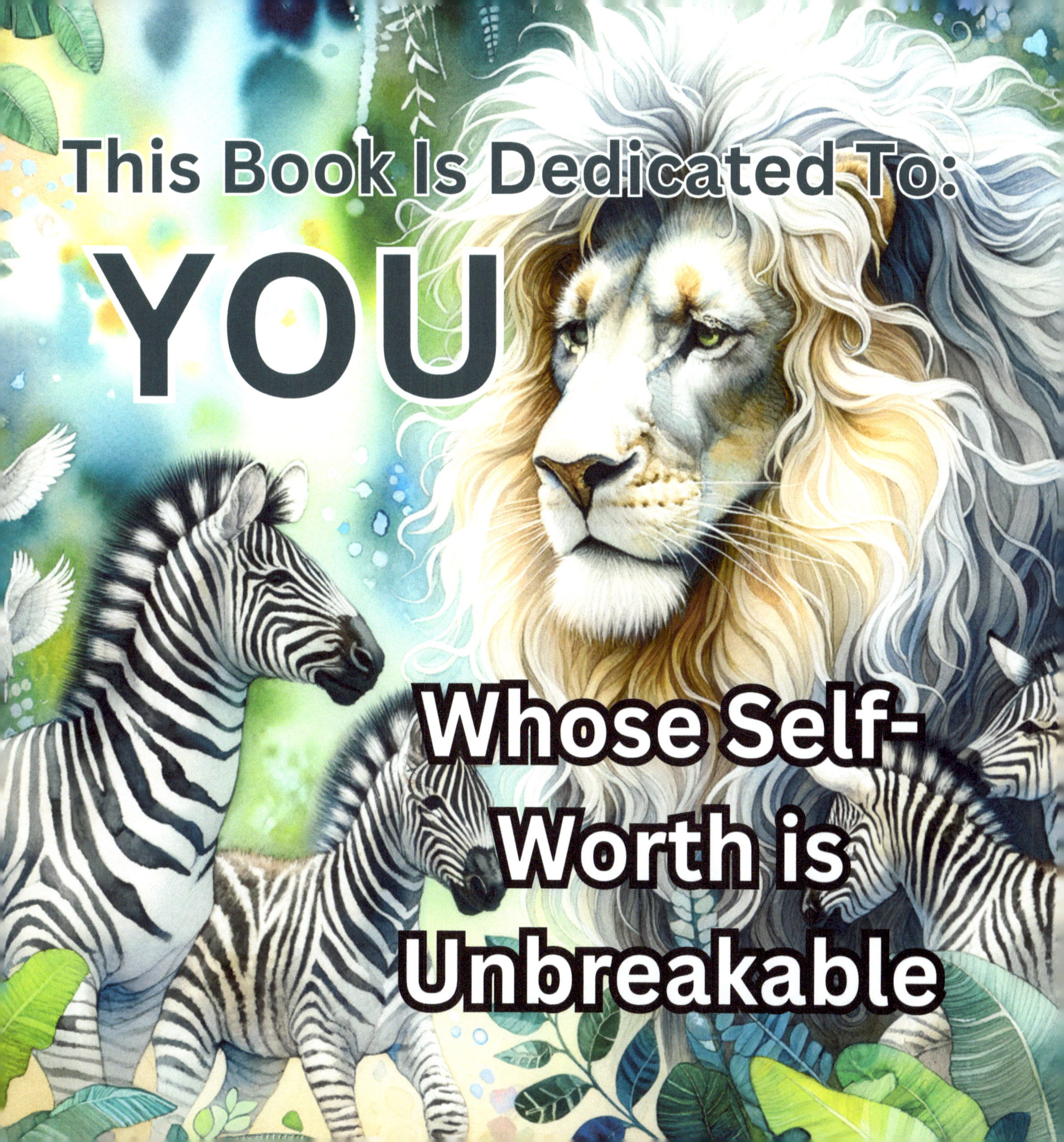

This Book Is Dedicated To:
YOU
Whose Self-Worth is Unbreakable

In the heart of the sunlit Silver Hills, where the grass whispers secrets to the breeze, old Leo the lion lay under his favorite baobab tree.

His mane gleamed like the golden sun, but today, his majestic face looked as stormy as a raincloud.

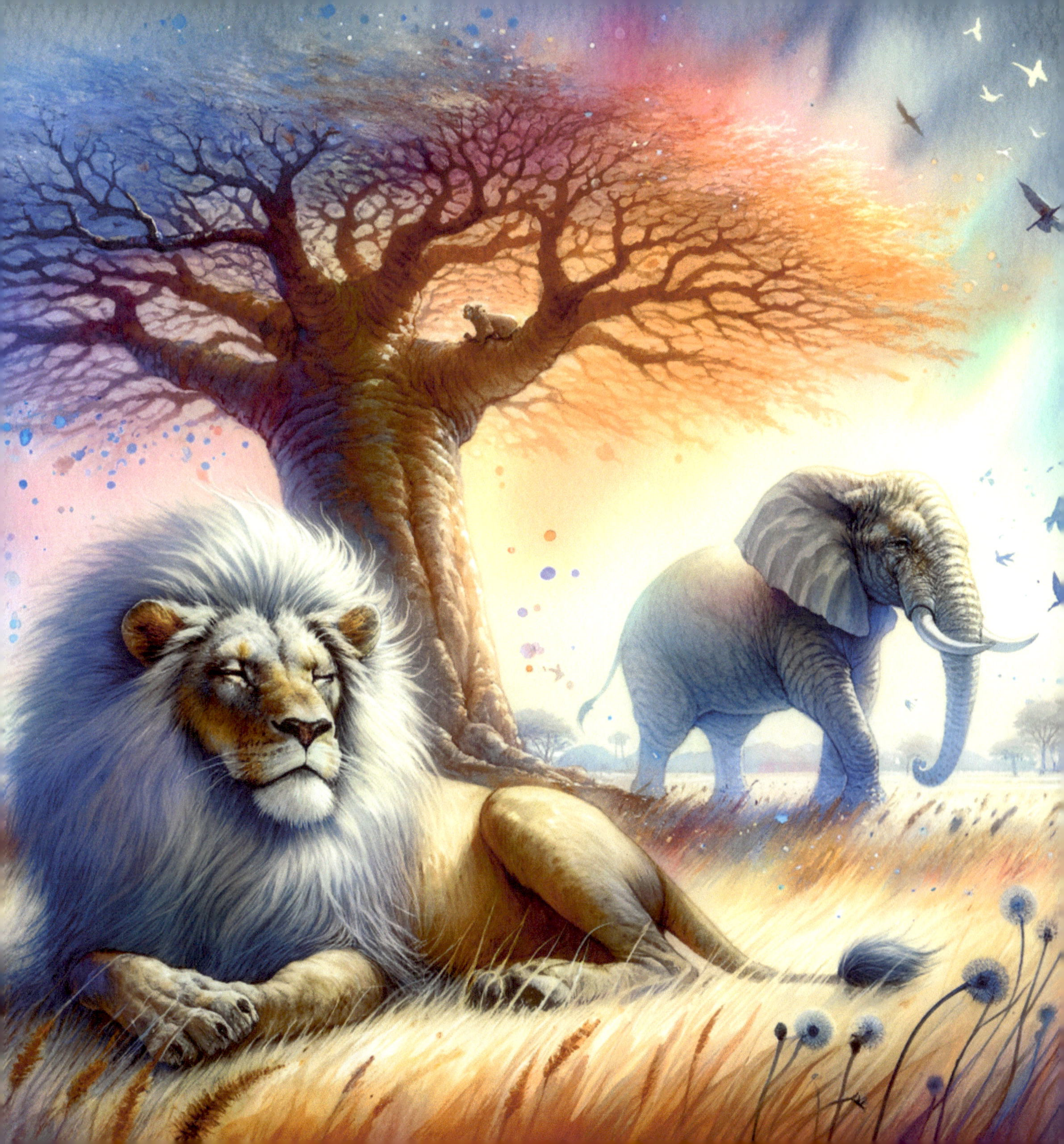

Nearby, Ed the wise old elephant lumbered over, his great ears flapping like the wings of a giant bird.

"Why the long face, Leo?" Ed asked with a twinkle in his gray, wrinkled eyes.

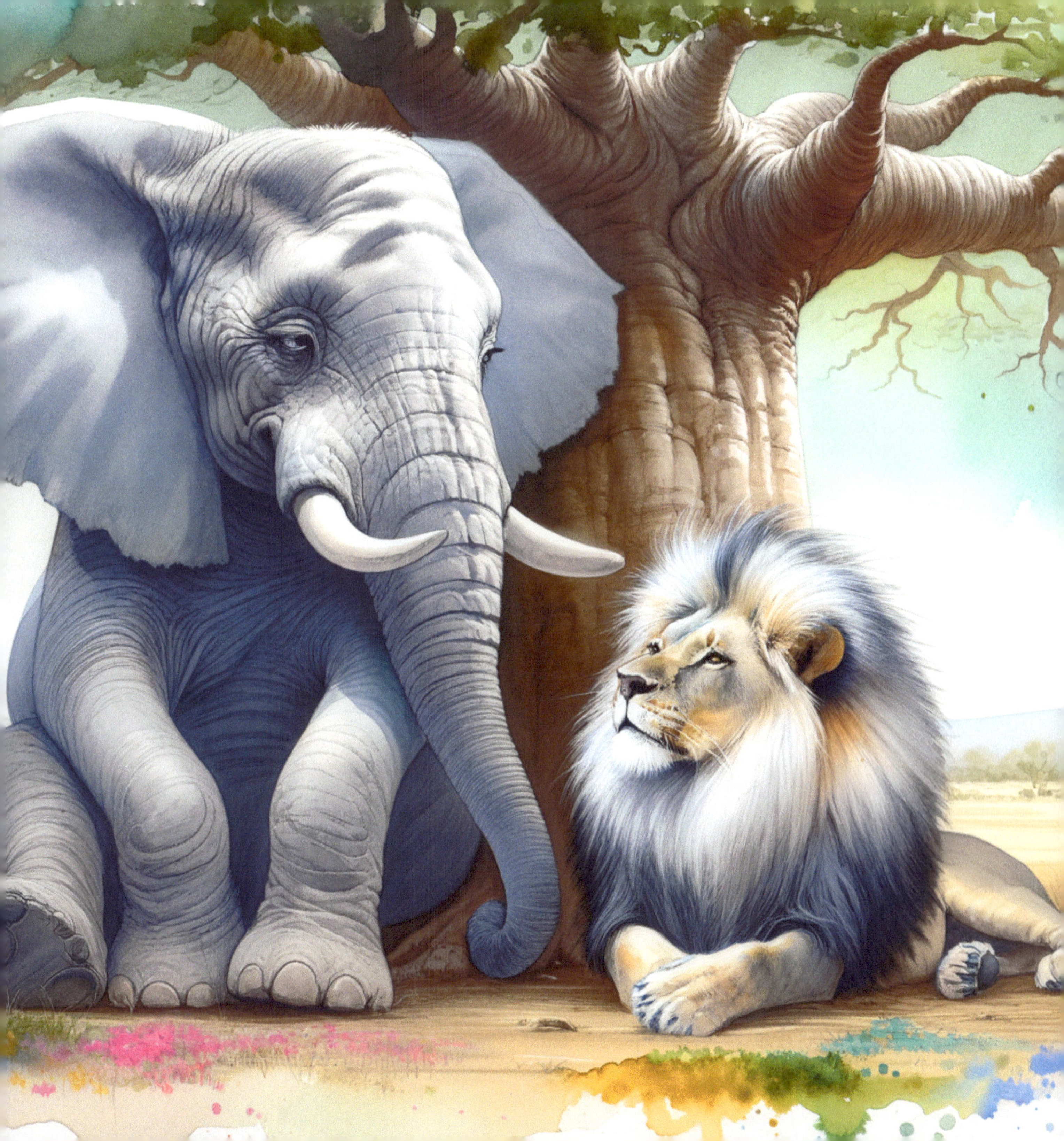

Leo sighed, "Oh Ed, today the monkeys called me 'slow' and 'grumpy.'

It made me feel small, like a mouse instead of the King of the Jungle."

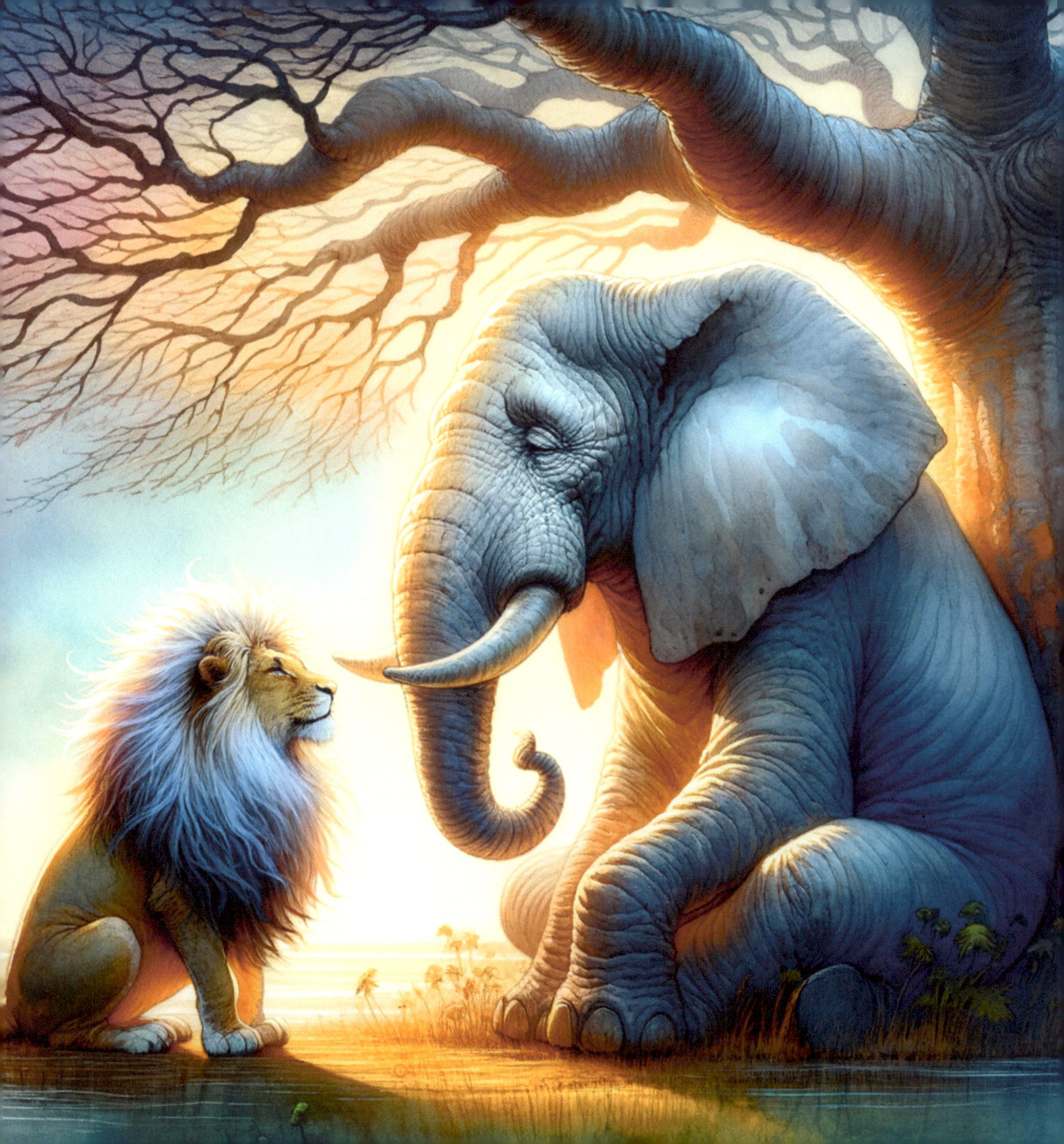

Ed nodded thoughtfully, tugging at the grass with his trunk. "Ah, words can sting, Leo.

But do you remember the Golden Light we talked about? It lives inside you, glowing with your true strength."

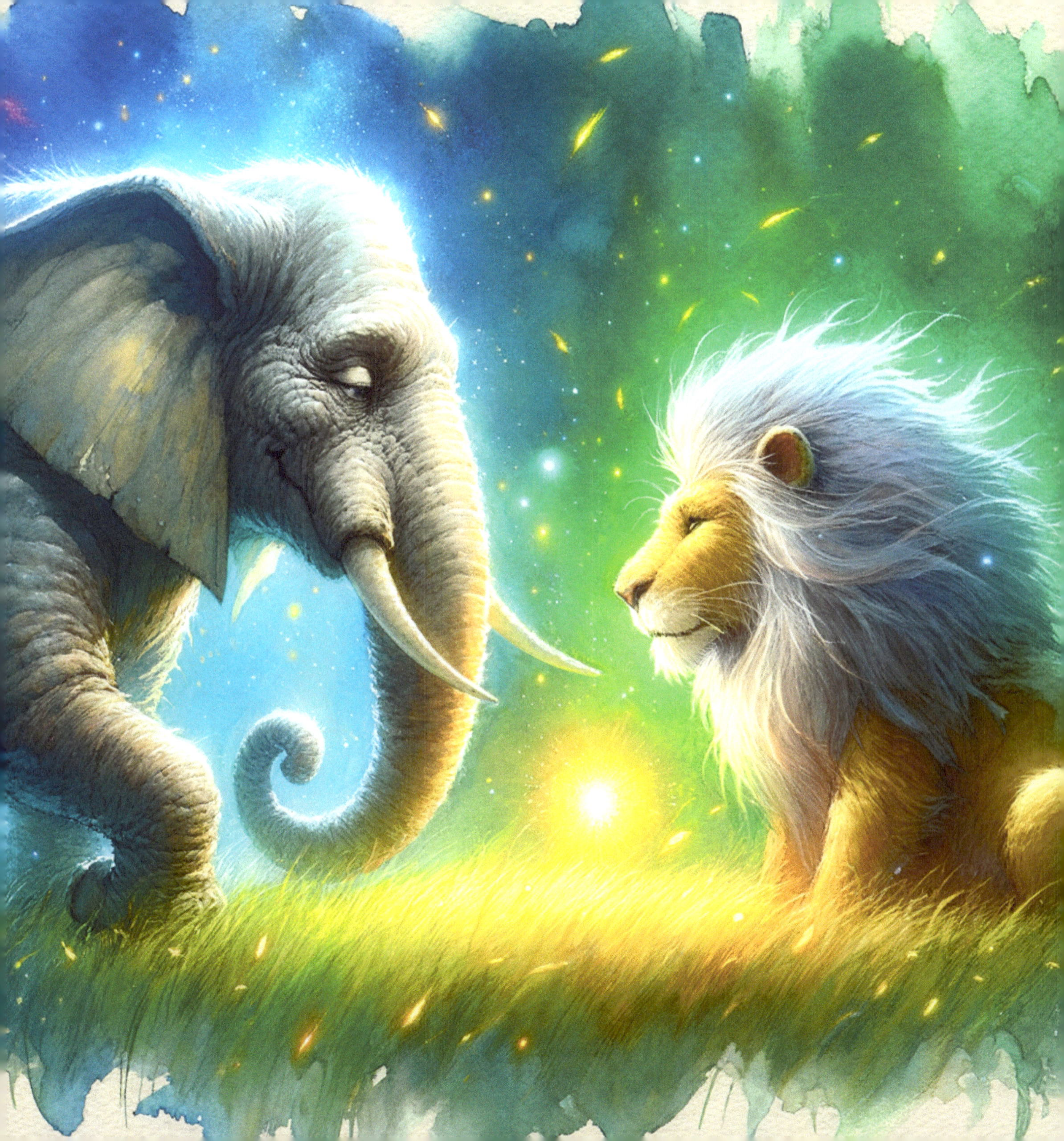

Leo's eyes sparkled with curiosity.

"But how can the Golden Light inside me help when others say such mean things?"

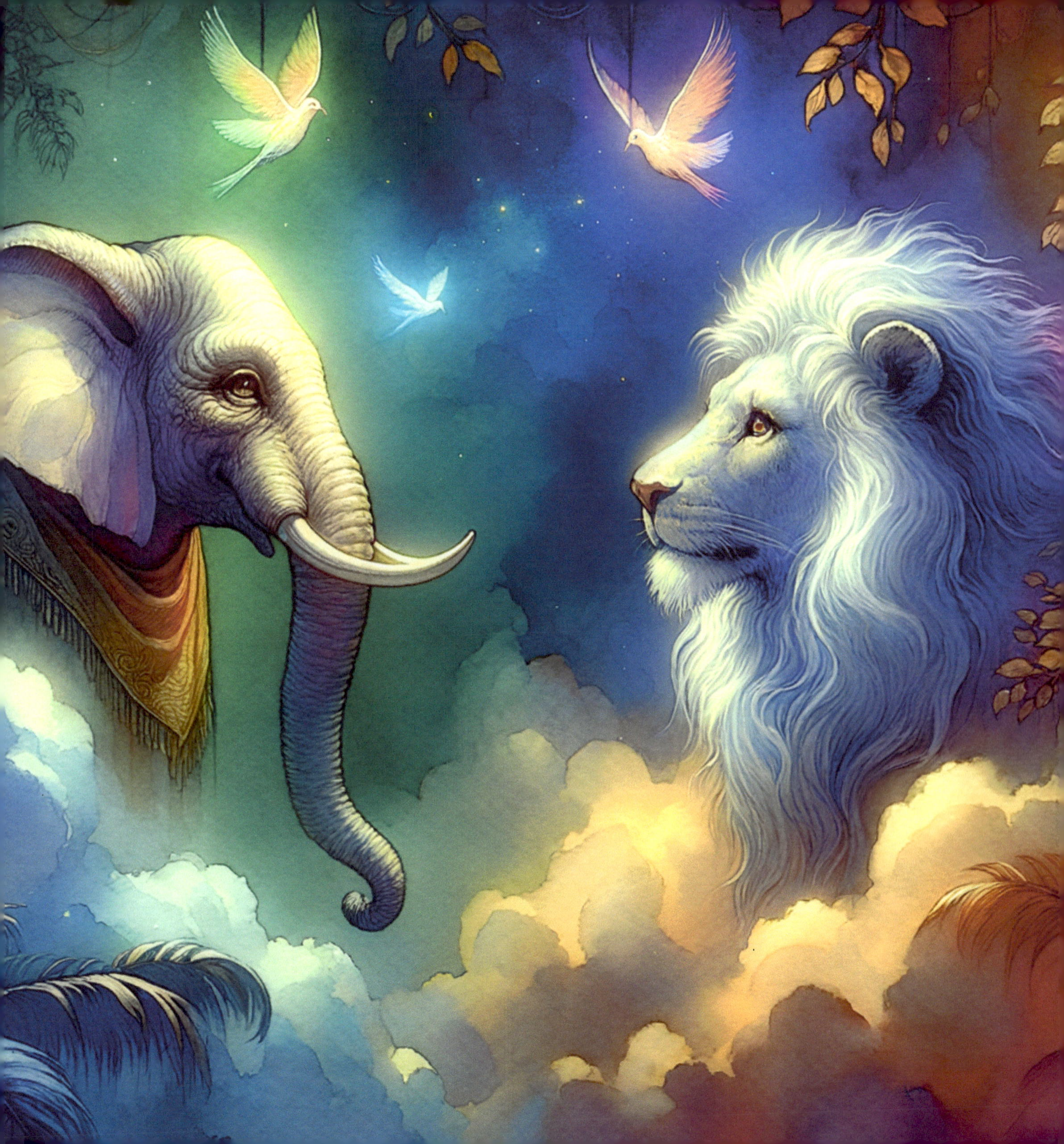

"Just like you choose not to pounce and roar," Ed explained, "you can choose not to let those words shake your big lion heart.

Your Golden Light—your kindness and wisdom—is your silent strength."

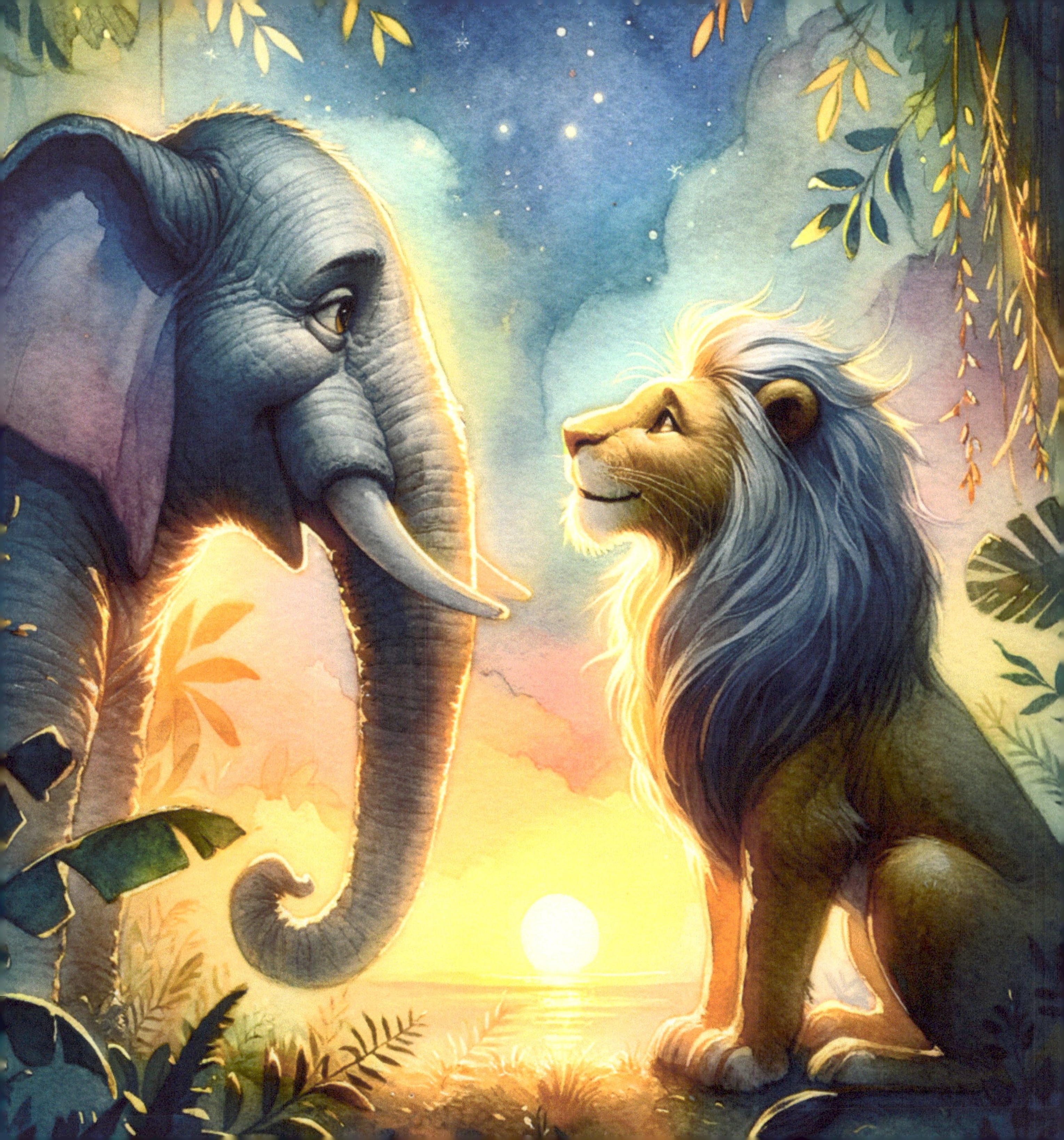

The next day, as Leo strolled through the Jungle, the zebras began to whisper and giggle.

"Here comes the slow King," they sneered.

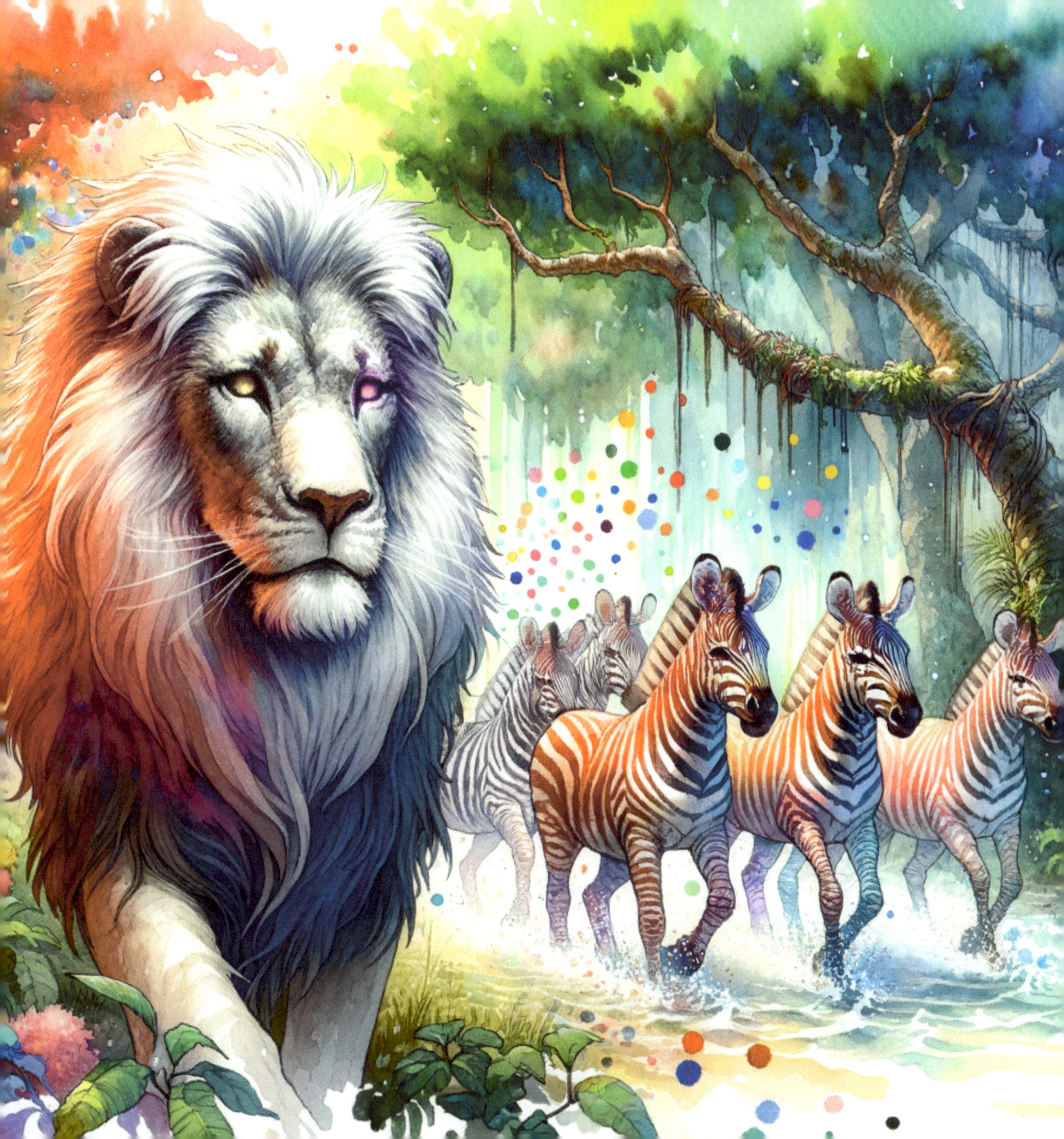

Leo felt a twinge in his heart but remembered the Golden Light.

Instead of growling, he simply smiled and waved his mighty paw. "Good day, speedy zebras," he said gently.

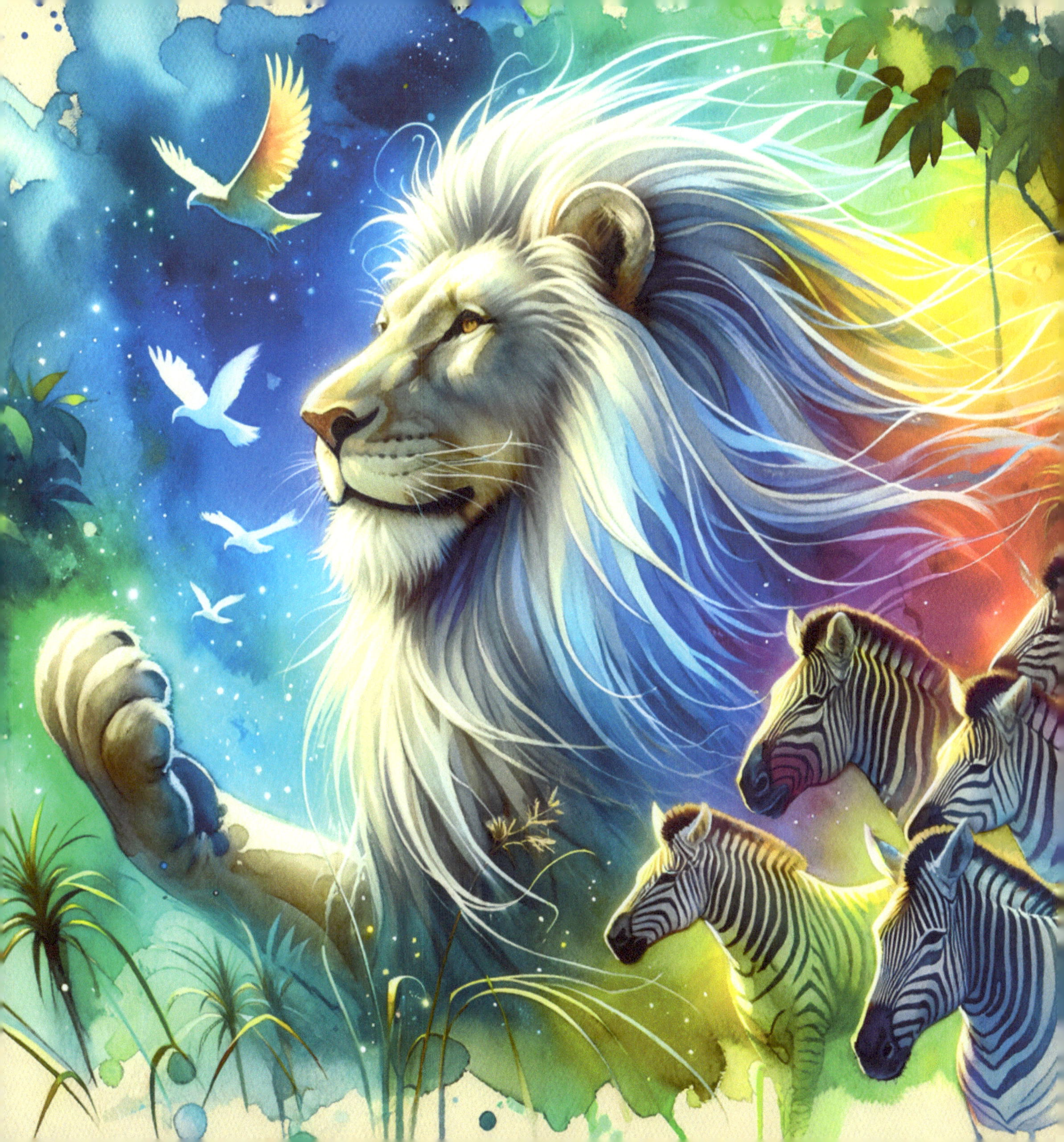

The zebras stopped giggling. They looked at each other, surprised by Leo's calm kindness.

One by one, their smiles returned, genuine and warm.

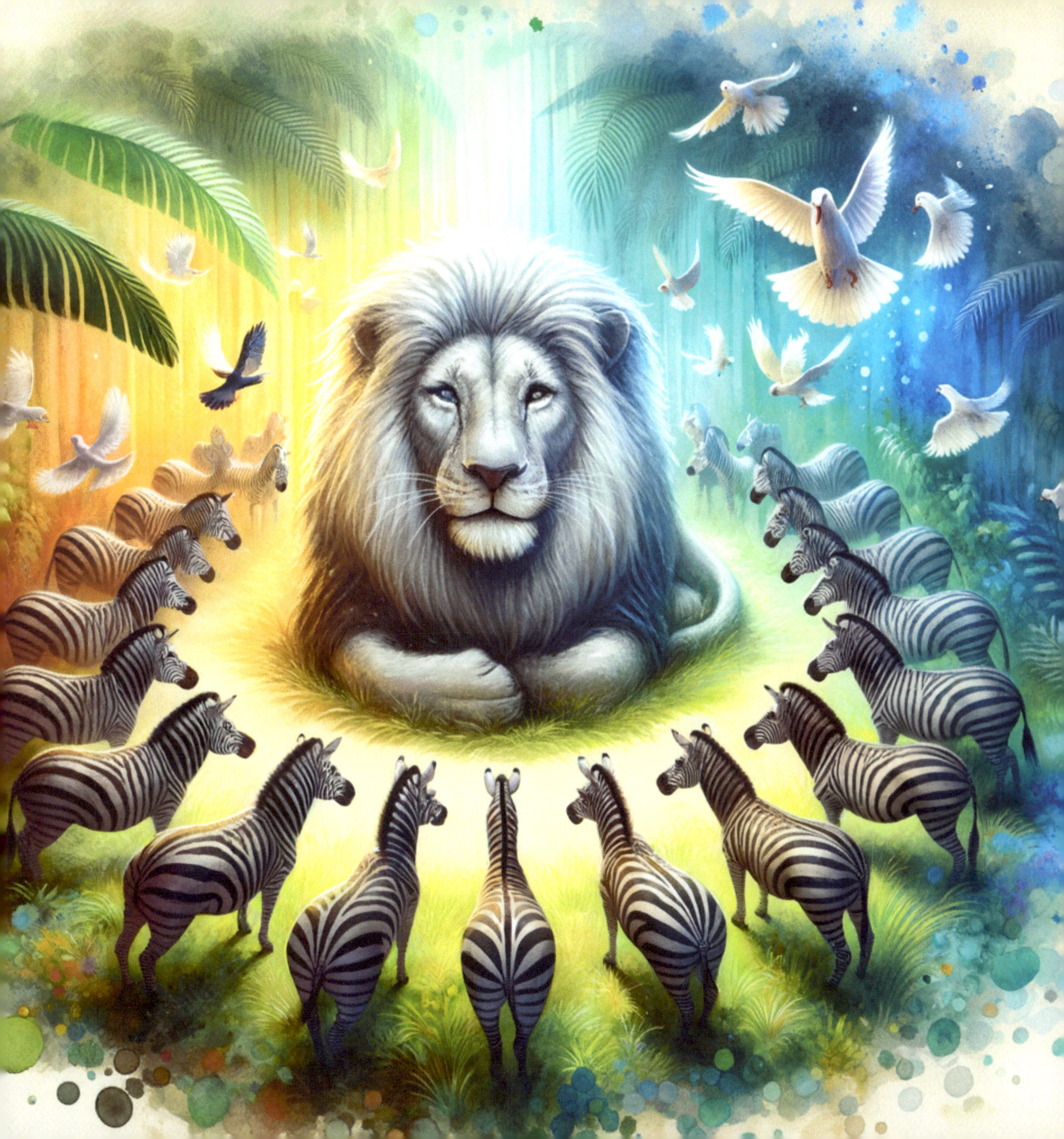

Later, under the cool shade of the baobab tree, Leo shared his encounters with Ed.

"I felt stronger, not showing my claws or teeth, just my heart," Leo admitted.

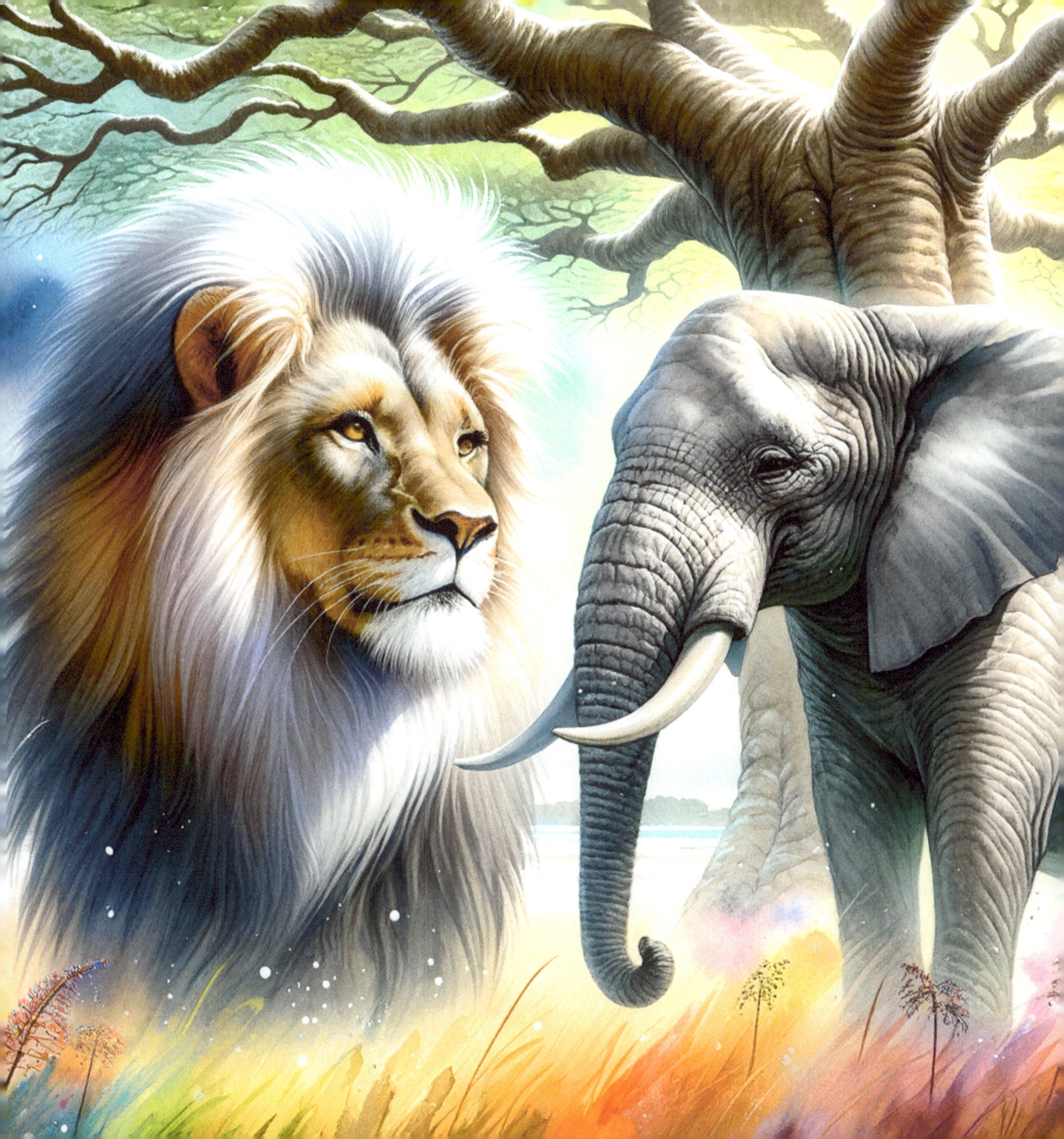

"Well done, Leo," Ed trumpeted. "You've discovered that true strength and power isn't about force;

it's about choosing peace, even when others do not."

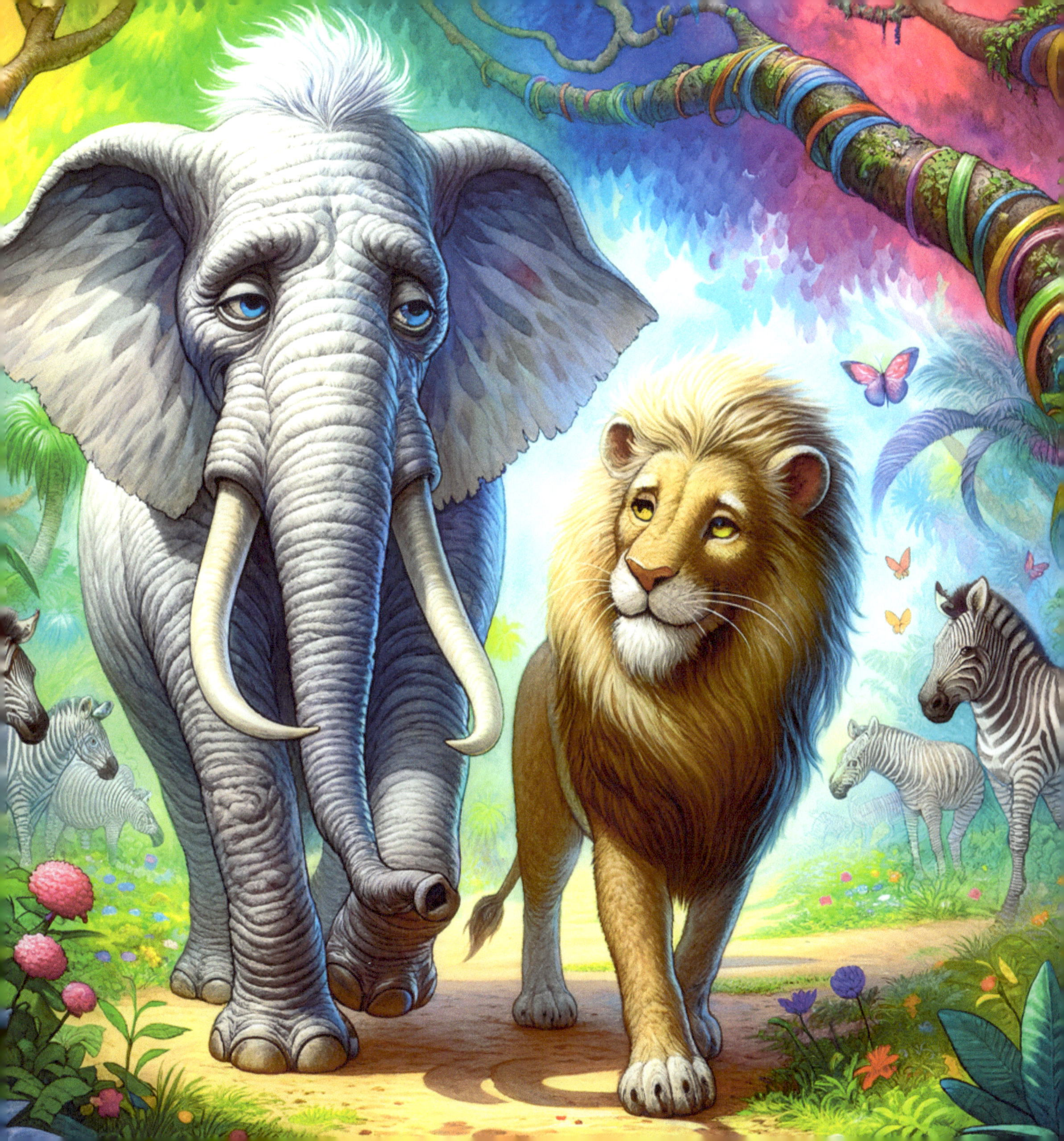

As the sun set, painting the sky with strokes of pink and orange, more animals from the Jungle came to sit near Leo, drawn by his gentle strength.

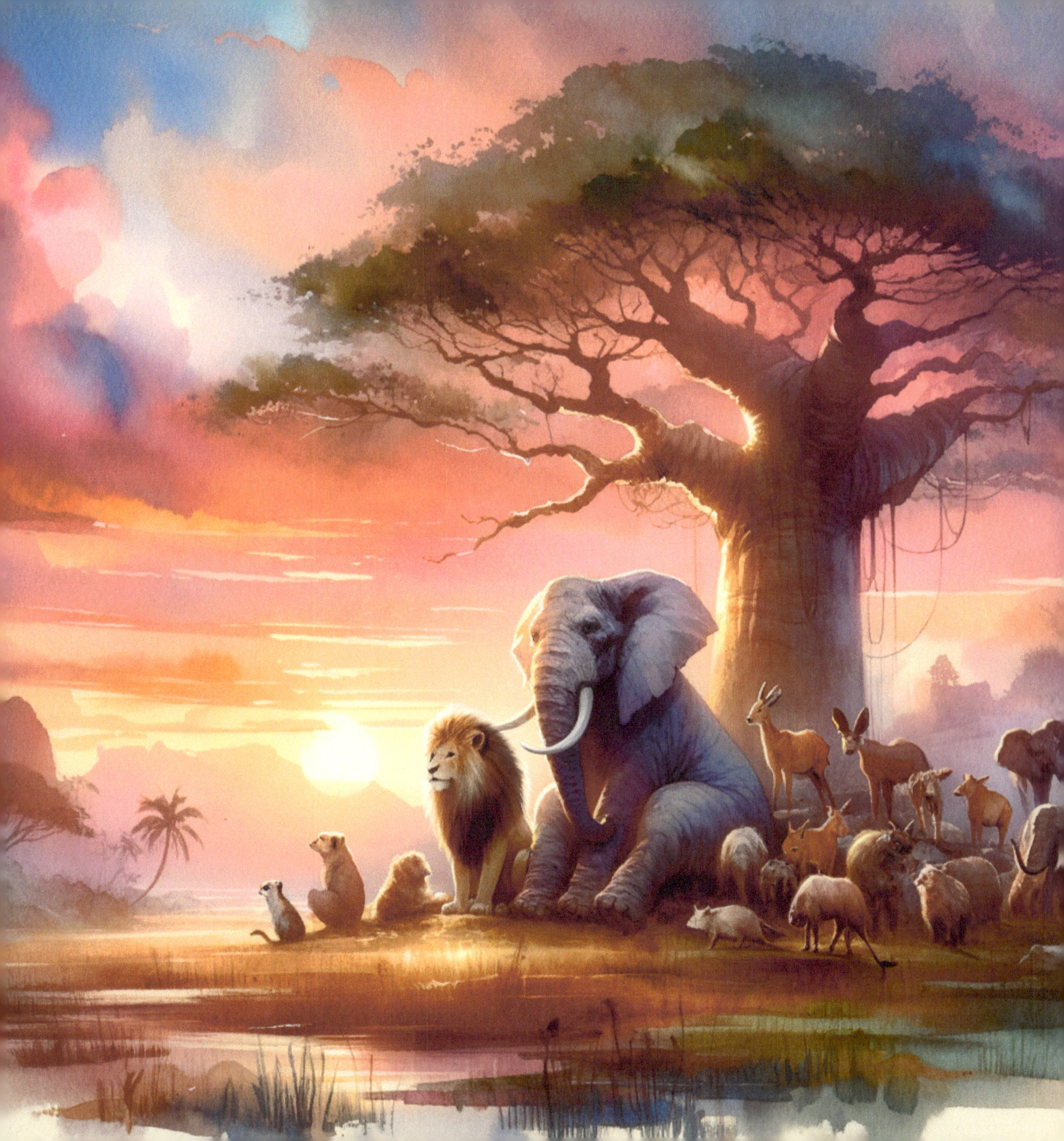

The whispers around Leo changed. "He truly is a wise King," said a giraffe.

"Yes, mighty not just in body but in spirit," added a caribou.

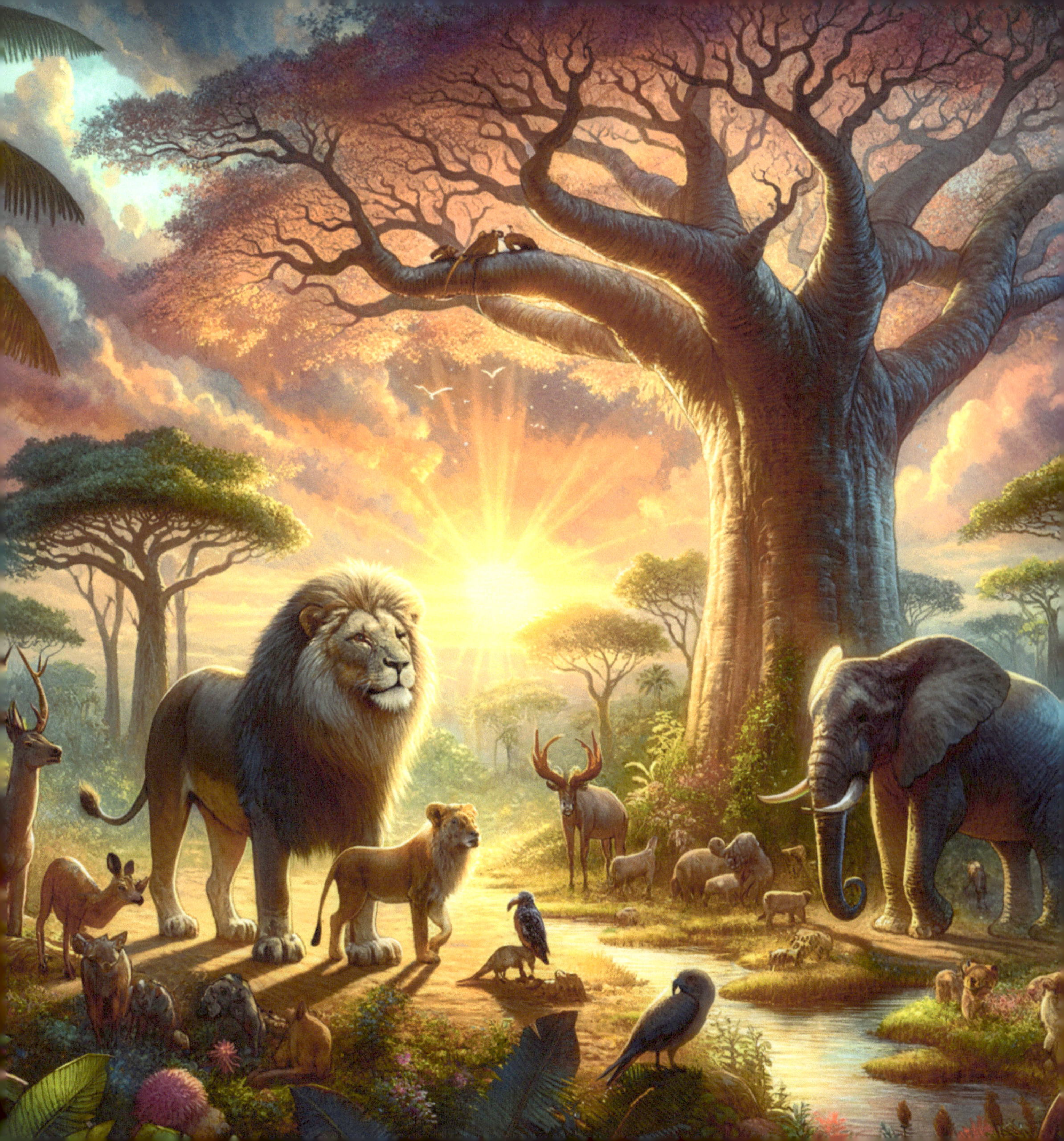

Leo's heart swelled with joy.

The Golden Light within him wasn't just his secret anymore—it was a beacon for all.

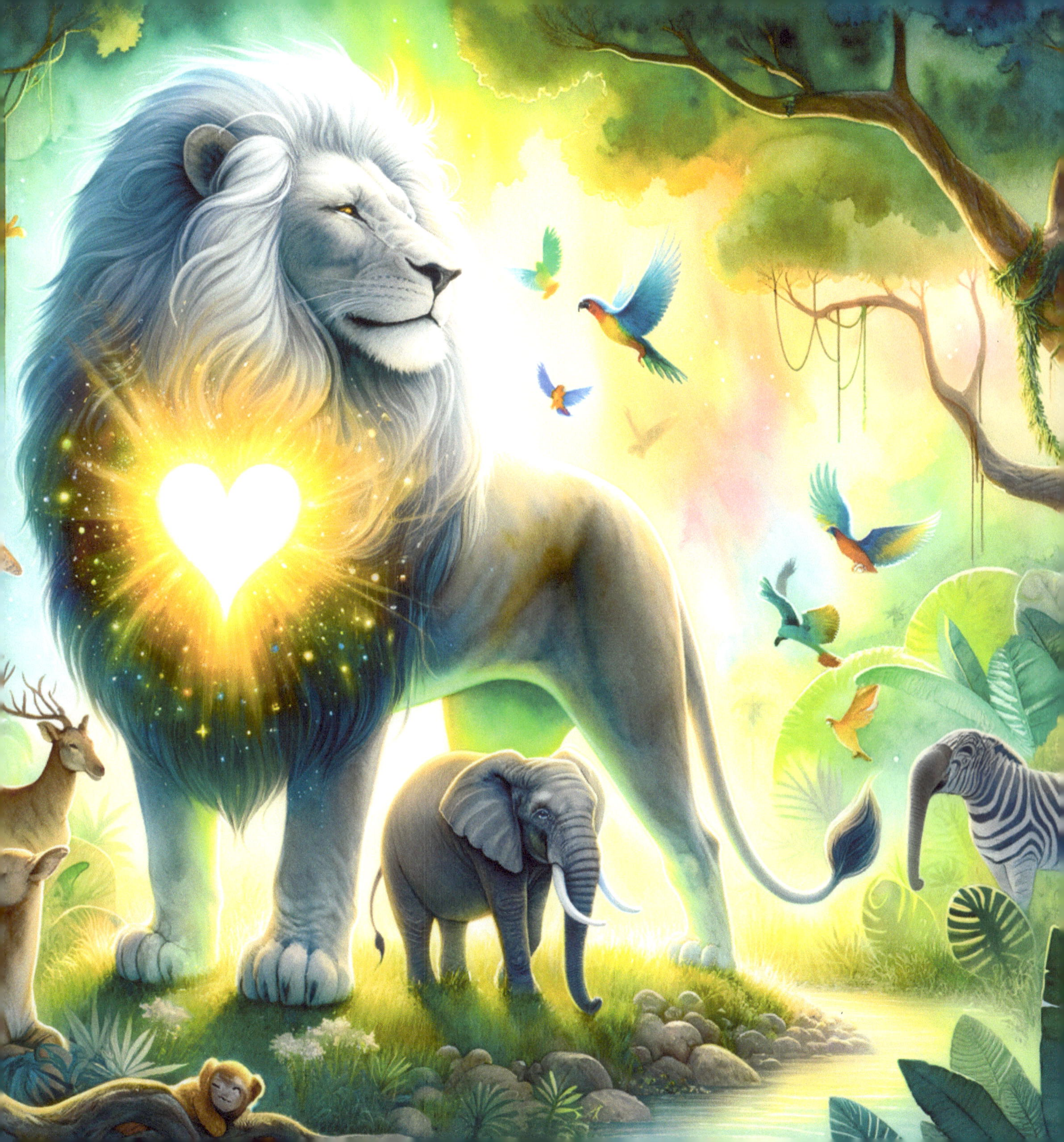

Ed smiled, his eyes gleaming with pride. "See, my friend?

Your silent strength—your Golden Light—touches everyone around you, more powerful than the loudest roar."

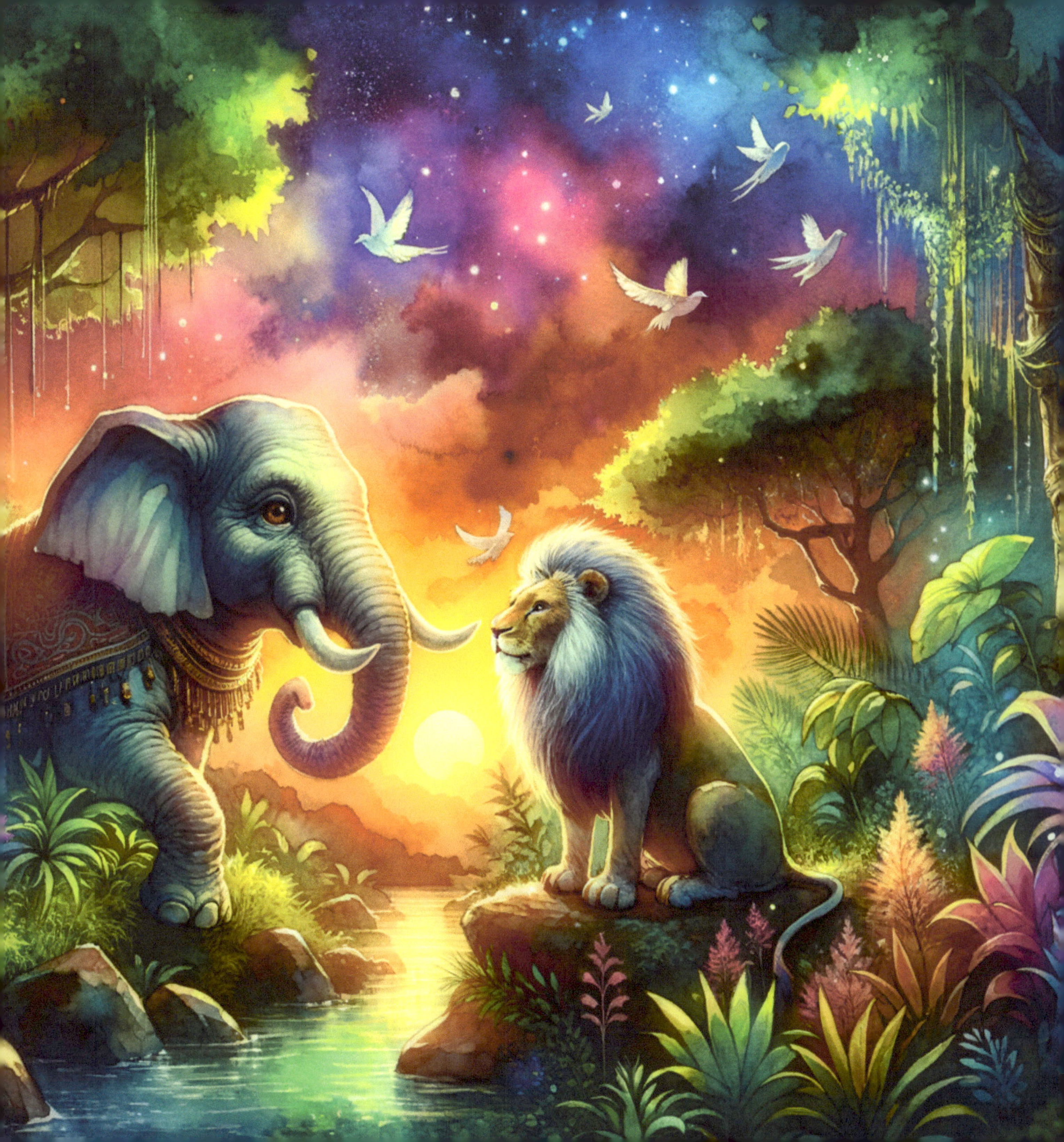

From that day on, Leo no longer feared the words of others.

With the Golden Light guiding him, he knew his true strength came from within, making him a King not just of the Jungle, but of his own heart.

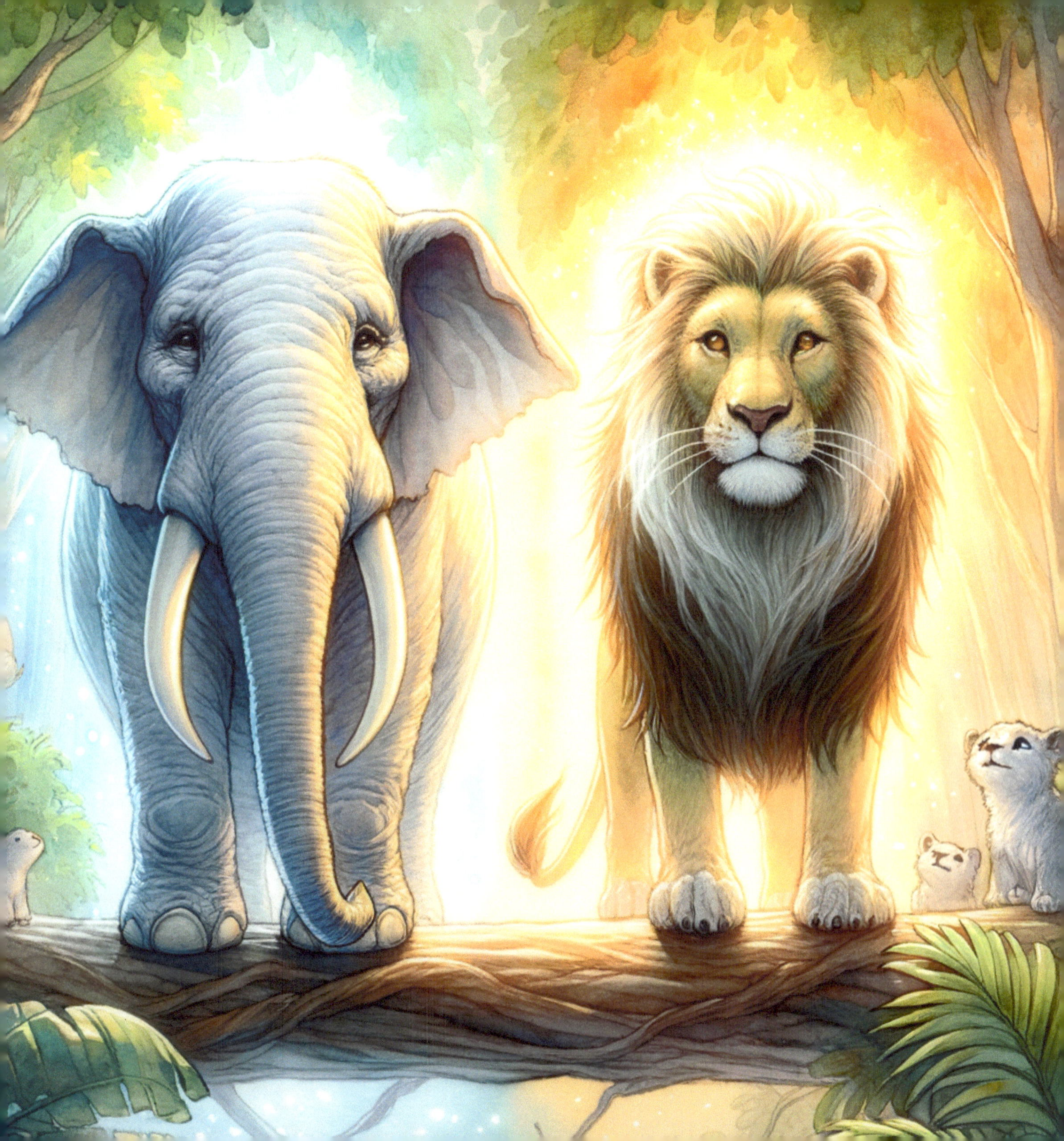

FOR YOUR ADULT COLORING BOOK PRINTABLE, SCAN QR CODE HERE:
FOR MORE BOOKS BY THIS AUTHOR, SCAN QR CODE HERE: